Ebola: 2015

LIVING THROUGH THE OUTBREAK.

By:
Marshal "ZB" Jacobs

I0428603

I dedicate this book to the people working day and night to ensure stories like this one remain on the fiction side of a very thin line.

Preface

With everything that is happening right now in the world, it seemed the time was right for someone to write a short story about Ebola that offers real tips and tricks to protect your family. There is no reason you shouldn't be able to enjoy a good story while you learn about protecting the people you love.

If you are like me then you would do anything to protect your family. I find there are different levels of security people strive for. Some will spare no expense to be prepared for whatever black swan event might happen. They believe this ensures the greatest chance of survival for their families. Others are much more skeptical and might rely on social order and good will to protect their families. As a father and husband, I believe putting your family in the care of social order or the government is a mistake of the gravest kind.

You may wonder why I chose to write a non-fiction book in fictitious form; Easy, many people get bored quickly with non-fiction books, so I like to add a story to otherwise boring facts and details about something. This helps keep the interest of whomever the audience happens to be.

With that said, I sat out to write this book to help my fellow human being. This might be a fiction book, but remember, it uses real principles practiced in homes and hospitals around the world. The first choice is always professional medical care, but if that is unavailable then utilize whatever gives you the best chance for survival.

Don't give up. You can protect your family from deadly viruses like Ebola. Learn how to keep yourself and your loved ones safe. Education is and always will be the most important tool in your survival arsenal.

Introduction

You will be walked through the life of a young professional writer as he discovers what it is like when Ebola comes close to home. Join him and Eva as they learn how to protect themselves and their living space from the constant threat lurking outside their door.

Randy and Eva take the time to build an elaborate cleaning station in the garage for whoever decided to leave and reenter. They improvised ways to clean their food before it entered their cupboard.

Take a ride on the coaster with Randy and Eva as they struggle to survive the constant threat of death by Ebola. This is your chance to find out what worked for them and what you might be able to do should you ever find yourself in a similar situation.

Though this book may be written as fiction it was based on actual practices used to keep people safe from viruses such as Ebola. Don't underestimate any of the viruses and diseases that threaten you and your family.

Take the time to learn what you can do in the event of an out of control epidemic. You owe that to yourself and your family.

November 3rd, 2014

When Randy woke up, he slowly peeled his head off the computer desk and wiped away the drool that had escaped while he was sleeping. The sunlight penetrated his eyes through the sheets nailed over the windows. It exposed the debris and dust that filled the room.

He rubbed his head, pulled a bottle of headache medicine from the pile of old soda cans, placed two pills in his mouth, and chased them down with the remnants of a drink from last night.

Randy clicked his mouse and began making his morning internet rounds. He checked his email, the news, and social media accounts. Finding nothing out of the ordinary other than an outbreak of Ebola in West Africa, he decided to grab some breakfast. Randy picked up a handful of trash from his desk and carefully walked it to the kitchen trashcan before washing his hands, grabbing some breakfast and a can of soda, and heading back to his computer.

Upon return to the computer he noticed Eva was online and started a chat with her. "Morning, Eva." He messaged.

Eva replied, "Is it morning already? I guess I've been working on this new website at the CDC for over 30 hours."

Randy responded, "Don't overdo it." Then he asked, "Hey, I was going to hit the grocery store at 4th and Young tonight, if you would like to join me. You've been saying you want to see this place. You want to meet me there? Say, six or seven tonight?"

She didn't immediately respond. Several tense moments passed before she said, "Yeah, I'm game, but I'll be stuck at this computer until after seven. How about we meet around eight?"

"That sounds great." He responded.

Eva replied, "Okay. Now, unless you want to talk about the new Ebola site for the CDC, I need to get back to work."

"See you tonight." He said before closing out the chat window.

Randy looked at his handwritten poster-board schedule hanging on the wall and popped open his soda can. His project deadline was fast approaching, but he had barely started. He stretched, rubbed his hands through his strawberry-blonde hair, and placed his fingers on the keyboard and began working on his new book.

The next 4 hours composed of one long trancelike state of typing, clicking, and researching. When he snapped out of it and looked away from the screen, Randy realized it was already five o'clock. He took a quick break to grab some lunch and a shower.

When he sat back down at the computer, he went through his normal rounds of checking his email, the news, and social media. Nothing major going on, some skirmishes in the Middle East, and the Ebola outbreak had officially reached the death toll of five thousand.

Unable to find his 'zone' again to continue writing, Randy picked up his phone, wallet, and keys and headed for the front door. He walked out into a nice suburban neighborhood on the edge of the city; the perfect location for raising a family. Randy made his way over to his rusty old blue truck, opened the creaky door, got in, and headed to the grocery store to meet Eva.

He arrived to the parking lot of what appeared to be a very old supermarket. The doors were made of wood and swung from hinges like the old Wild West saloon doors. There were barrels of fruits and vegetables stacked around the entrance. Even the neon sign looked antique. Randy got out of his truck, walked up to the entrance, and sat down on an old bench to wait for Eva.

She arrived at precisely eight o'clock. Randy didn't expect any less from her. She seemed to always have everything down to the smallest detail. She looked like the girl next door. Eva was the kind of woman that would be as happy rolling around in the mud as she would be in formal attire at the opera. Her blue-jeans contoured around her curves while her blouse complemented her hazel eyes and brunette hair. When she got to Randy, they greeted each other and walked inside.

"Wow, you're right." Eva said as she grabbed his sleeve. "This place is huge."

Randy leaned into her and said, "Didn't I tell you? Oh, and the prices are great, too." He pulled her toward the produce section.

Eva stopped him. There was obviously something on her mind. "Can I ask you a question?" She said.

"Of course." He responded.

She started talking about Ebola and what she had heard and learned in the past few weeks. "You know I've been contracted to work on the CDC website. I've worked around and talked to some very smart people at the CDC. You could say I've made some friends. Well, from what we've spoken about with Ebola, this virus is very dangerous. It broke five thousand killed and eight thousand infected this week. We could have a million person outbreak or worse within six months." She paused.

Randy looked at her sort of stunned and replied, "Okay. What is your question? And, how bad is this outbreak going to be? Should we be worried?"

Eva confided, "I'm not sure that we should be worried, yet. Though, I was hoping you and me could talk about what we would do to prepare for the possibility of an outbreak happening here?" She said with a persuasive flow to her voice.

"Why not?" He questioned. "Where do you want to start?"

She began talking like she had rehearsed the entire speech, "If things get really bad, we will need to create some clean area where we can shelter in place. You live on the edge of town, so I think the sterile area should be your home. We are going to need a clean way to enter and exit, so your garage would be converted into a cleaning room. Basically, the entrance into the house would go through the garage." She paused a moment to think before continuing, "First, there will be a room where all clothing can be stripped and placed into a washing machine with bleach. This room will also have a large sink we can use to dip canned goods and fresh produce in before taking it into the house. Then there will be a shower where we will use antibacterial soap to wash our bodies before entering the home. After that is another clothing room with a washing machine and dryer. Last comes the living quarters, which require special precautions of their own be taken."

He interjected, "We might need to write some of this down…"

"We will." She interrupted. "The inside will need to be stocked with enough food and water to last us at least several months. The more we have available the better. We could start building that supply today." She said.

"Hold on." Randy replied. "When did this go from just talking about it to actually living it?"

She raised an eyebrow and put on her cutest face before saying, "In light of recent events and information I have obtained, which I cannot share with you… I think it is a very good idea for us to start preparing now." Then she sat in a sheepishly coy position and waited for his answer.

"You really think this is going to get bad?" He asked.

"Yes. Sadly, I think it is going to get very bad." She said. "Let me explain. The new website I've been working on for the CDC is all about protecting yourself and your family during an outbreak. The people I've been working with are pretty certain this thing is going to last a long time and kill a lot of people. Ebola kills between twenty-five and ninety percent of the people who are infected. Forecast models show current growth rates of infected people will reach a peak in mid to late 2015. Before February of 2015 we could have well over a million deaths from Ebola with thousands of new and untreated cases every day. It could peak out near a billion deaths by mid 2016. That's about one in six people on earth!"

"Eva." He said. "That's got to be wrong. You're talking about almost 20% of all people. Why hasn't anyone said anything? I've been reading the papers. They say everything is under control."

She put her hand on his shoulder and said, "They're worried it will cause a panic that could kill more people than the epidemic."

He questioned her with disbelief, "What? Are you kidding me?"

"I'm afraid not. This is real." She told him.

Randy looked around the grocery store and pondered what it would be like to lose one in six people. He considered the panic that would ensue from such a tragedy. Then, he pondered the broken supply chains and command structures of governments. It all sounded pretty bad. "We've got to warn people." He said.

"It won't work." She told him. "The CDC will call you crazy and get you locked up. They don't want this thing getting out. They've been preparing to sustain themselves and a select number of government functions through the epidemic."

He responded, "We have to try, Eva. We have to try."

"Fine." She said. "Write a blog about it and share it with your friends and family. If it catches on, so be it. When it doesn't catch on, at least you'll have tried to warn everyone. Just don't try going on one of those conspiracy shows on TV or anything."

"Deal." He said. "Now, you said something about stocking up on food, right?" Randy asked.

"Yes, that's right." She replied with a brief pause before continuing, "Let's begin stocking up on staples like enriched dry rice, dried beans, salt, canned meats, and canned fruits and vegetables. It's also a good idea to stock up on drinking water, medical supplies, toiletries, and bleach."

"I think we are going to need another cart." He said as he walked back toward the entrance, returning moments later with two extra shopping carts. "We fill one with canned goods, one with medical supplies and toiletries, and the other one with water and dry rice and beans. Would that be a good start?" He asked her.

Eva smiled and said, "I think it is a great beginning to a lot of preparations we are going to do over the next few months. But, you forgot about bleach. That is a crucial component to keeping ourselves safe."

"Okay. The bleach goes on the bottom of the toiletries and medical supplies cart. You get all that and I'll grab the food and water?" He asked.

"Let's do it." She said as she pulled the cart from him and headed toward medical supplies. While walking away she looked over her shoulder and shouted, "Meet you back here in about thirty minutes."

He agreed and they both went through the store filling their cart with goods. By the time thirty minutes had arrived they were both done and met at the checkout. Eva said, "I got a couple of cool things from the camping section, too." She paused for effect before continuing,

"We can take the truck back to your place and talk about how to convert the garage while we put everything away."

Randy responded with astonishment, "You really want to get this ball rolling fast, don't you?"

"If you'd seen and heard what I saw and heard then you'd be right here with me. You have to trust me." She pleaded.

"I trust you with my life." He said as he paid the tab for their little shopping extravaganza.

"You obviously trust me with your bank account." She said before asking, "Did we really spend fourteen-hundred dollars?"

"Yep, we sure did." He told her as he pushed the carts through the old wooden doors and toward his truck.

They loaded the groceries and agreed to call it a night. Since she had ridden the bus to the grocery store, Randy dropped Eva off at her place before he returned home to put away the supplies they picked up. He left the medical supplies in the bags for Eva to put away. That was really her department anyway. Once he finished, Randy sat down at his computer desk and went through the rounds to check his email, the news, and his social media. Nothing had really changed in the past few hours. He decided to write the blog post he spoke to Eva about before going to bed. After about an hour of writing he was ready to share his knowledge with his friends and family:

Preparing for the Coming Ebola Epidemic

Most of the people who read this post are going to blow it off and act like I am simply off-my-rocker. I'm not crazy, but I don't blame you for thinking I am. Honestly, I didn't believe what you are about to read either until a very close and trusted friend confided in me what she knew. You are welcome to take this information or leave it. I am not forcing your hand. Of course, I hope you take what I wrote and follow through. Even a little bit of prevention could save your life and the lives of your loved ones. Share it with your friends and family in hopes they will heed the advice and survive what some believe is to come.

Africa has now seen over five thousand deaths. Before February of 2015 we are expecting the death toll to reach over one million. You must protect your family. When the outbreak becomes a global epidemic it will be too late for you to prepare. You must begin now. Here is what you can do. Learn about how Ebola is contracted, protect yourself and your family from infection, practice safe procedures for anything that can result in exposure, and store enough supplies to get through any epidemic.

So, how is Ebola contracted? You can get Ebola from direct contact with the bodily fluids of an infected person or animal, dead or alive. These fluids include blood, semen, urine, saliva, vomit, feces, and even sweat. If these fluids come into contact with any cut, abrasion, or get into the mouth, nose, eyes, or sexual organs, you are likely to catch Ebola.

You can only catch this particular virus from someone or something that already shows the symptoms of Ebola: fever, severe headache, muscle pain, weakness, diarrhea, vomiting, abdominal pain, and unexplained bleeding or bruising. The symptoms can begin to show themselves from 2 days after infection to as long as three weeks after infection.

Once you understand the threat, it is time to protect yourself from Ebola. You should setup a clean-room and write a safety plan for what you and your family will do in the event of an outbreak. This plan should include a way to clean foods and equipment of the virus, wash your clothes in bleach, and wash your bodies with antibacterial soap. This should all be in a room separate from the living area. A garage works great for this. My plan is to build a shower in my garage right by the door leading into the house. Before that will be a large sink for soaking goods in bleach-water and a washing machine for washing my clothes with bleach-water.

Protecting yourself from the contagion with a layer barrier when you are in an infected zone, and ensuring you clean that barrier layer with bleach, and clean everything you are taking in, including yourself, you can better protect your family from Ebola. Because the virus is not airborne, it is much harder to contract when you follow these precautions. Wear gloves when you go shopping in a hot-zone. Cover as much of your body as you can comfortably cover with a protective layer meant to keep bodily fluids of infected people from spreading to you and your family. Anyone that enters a hot-zone for any reason should not share a bathroom or bed with those not at risk. Maintain strict cleanliness standards and use bleach regularly to clean everything from fresh fruit to tools, dishes, or clothes. Ebola has a hard time living outside of the human body.

Don't forget one of the most important factors in the event of an emergency: If you store enough food, water, and supplies to last the entire cycle of the epidemic, then you won't have to worry about risking exposure by going out during the crisis to get supplies.

Spend the next several months stocking up on food and water for you and your family. Try *and buy supplies that you already use. I'm working up to a two year supply of essential foods, medical supplies, and toiletries. This gives me enough time to rotate through them before they expire. The food supplies can be tricky if you are on a tight budget, but over time you can store enough stock for months. Start with a on month supply and move on to a two month supply and so on until you reach a six month supply. This is a good short term stock in the event an epidemic like Ebola breaks out.*

Long term food should be a consideration once the short term supply has been established. My research shows food with a long shelf life is usually freeze-dried or powdered and sealed into foil packages or cans with inert gasses to stop bacterial growth. This supply can grow to as large as a 25 year shelf life allows.

No matter what you choose to do, as my friend, at least take these things into consideration. Avoid contact with any bodily fluid and clean your hands regularly with antibacterial soap or alcohol sanitizer. Ensure you clean foods brought home from any hot-zone. This is easily done by a quick spray with a bleach solution or a dip in a bleach-water bath. Be careful and be watchful. Your life and that of your family and friends is in your hands. Stay safe and be well.

Once it was posted to his website, Randy shared the new blog on all his social media sites and emailed it to a few of his close friends. After he finished his good deed for the night, he crawled his way to the bed in his room and fell onto the sheets. He passed out before he even had time to think about everything that had happened since he woke from his computer desk slumber.

December 31st, 2014

Eva walked into the kitchen at Randy's house and said, "Did you hear the news? The CDC says they think they've found a treatment. They are going to start inoculating infected people immediately."

Randy looked up from his book and replied, "Seriously? Do they think it's going to work? There are thousands of infected people in the United States alone. This could save so many lives."

"Well, my friend at the CDC says they ran human trials last week with a 100% success rate." Eva replied. "They should be done producing enough inoculations for everyone in the United States this week. Apparently, they are going to be giving the medication out to the worst cases first and go down the line. They are working with other countries to produce enough for the whole world." She told him.

He responded, "That is great news, but until it's over I'll continue to take precautions. Speaking of which, I've got to go to the store to pickup some food. I'm going to need your help when I come back. Is there anything you need me to get for you?"

Eva thought about asking him not to go, but didn't want him to stop her from going to the web programmers show that was coming up. So, instead of asking him not to go, she wrote him a small list: bleach, fruit, ground beef, chicken, hand sanitizer, and a few more spray bottles.

Randy took the list and began to "suit up." He replaced all of his clothing with thick white material that had been sprayed with water repellent. This kept fluids from accumulating on the fibers or seeping through them onto the wearer. Once he had everything on he made his way through the garage to the outside world. Aside from the clothing he wore a pair of sunglasses to protect his eyes, gloves to protect his hands, and carried a bottle of hand sanitizer and a small spray bottle of bleach-water.

When he arrived at the store, everyone was dressed to a different level of protection. Some people believed "the cure" was already here and they no longer needed to protect themselves, others cut down their protection a little, and some stayed very well protected. All the employees were wearing hazmat gear, and the entire store smelled like bleach. Randy made his way through and got what he needed. Luckily, they had everything on his list. This is the first time that has happened in a while.

He paid for the supplies and headed back to the house. When he got home he called out to Eva and asked her if she was ready to start the entrance procedure, "Eva, I'm back. Are you ready?"

Eva called back through the walls, "Ready for stage one."

"I'm coming in." He told her as he blocked the door open and began to bring the groceries inside. Randy stopped at the door and set the bags down on the floor. He looked at Eva and asked, "Is the bleach bath ready?"

"Yeah, it's there. Five Gallons of 0.5% chlorine solution just like what we use in our spray bottles." She said as she pointed to a large sink full of water.

He began the process of soaking the groceries, one by one, in the bleach solution and then placing them onto the adjacent table to dry. "Don't forget we have to wash these off after they dry to make sure there isn't any bleach residue left behind. Don't want to get sick." He said.

When he finished, he placed the store bags outside in the trashcan and then placed all of his clothing, shoes, underwear, hat, and everything else into the washing machine. He turned the washer on and poured in a cup of bleach. Then he walked under the shower and proceeded to scrub his body with antibacterial soap from the head down.

Once he was clean, she passed him a towel through the door. Randy wrapped the towel around his waist and stepped into the next level clean-room. This one had a washer and dryer and also smelled like bleach. Randy grabbed some clothes off of the washing machine and put them on before walking into the living area. Eva stuck her head in the clean-room and sprayed some bleach-water on the floor and around the washer and dryer.

"Did you get everything?" She asked him.

"Of course I got everything." He replied as he leaned back in his black reclining chair with a smirk.

"Good." She said. "I was going to pull out some games for later. You want to play chess?"

"Not tonight." He replied. "I was going to do some work on my new book."

Then Eva said, "By the way, I'm going to go to that web developer summit tomorrow. I'll need you to help me get back in when I return. Okay?"

Randy turned to her and sounded surprised, "The summit will have lots of people. More than six percent of the U.S. already has Ebola. There are bound to be infected people there. It isn't worth the risk."

She responded, "I'm going. This is for my career. I know your book career has taken off since this all started, but I still have to network for business. I'll be careful."

"I still think it's a bad idea, but I'll help you get back in." He told her as he made his way to the computer desk. Once they finished talking he began to go through the rounds of checking his email, the news, and his social media. The death toll had almost reached a quarter of a million. Randy called out, "Eva, death toll almost reached 250,000 people. They say another 60,000 are infected but seeking treatment."

She called to him from the kitchen, "I hope this is all finally behind us. I can't wait to go back to normal and stop worrying about everyone I love."

"Hopefully it is." He said. "Hopefully."

The rest of the night went smooth. Like they had each night before, they went to bed in separate rooms of the house, both at eight o'clock in the evening. The streets were much quieter at night now that no one wanted to go out and risk infection. It was almost peaceful.

January 24th, 2015

The past week has brought tragedy to the entire world. The inoculation we have been producing only placed the virus into hibernation. Little did we know, the virus was contagious during the dormant period. It is now believed that more than a half of a million people might be infected.

Eva wasn't downstairs for breakfast like she had been every morning at nine o'clock. Worried about her, he went to her door and knocked. "Eva, you okay."

"No. Stay out. I think I may have contracted the flu at the web developer summit." She tried to convince herself.

Randy got real serious, "You don't have the symptoms do you?"

She replied, "Well, fatigue, headache, fever, chills, feeling nauseous." She paused. "All of those. Just stay out of my room and sanitize anything you can. Keep me hydrated and make damn sure you don't get any of my fluids on you or in the house. It could just be the flu, or it could be Ebola."

"Eva." He said as he held back tears. "I can't lose you, Eva."

She joked, "I don't want you to lose me either."

Randy replied leaning against her door, "I don't think you understand. I think I love you, Eva."

She replied, "Don't say things like that right now. Save it for when I'm feeling better in a few days. Just take the precautions and follow the procedures we setup."

He agreed and went downstairs to get the necessary equipment to take care of her. Over the next several hours he setup a clean-room between her room and the rest of the house.

This room was made out of old plastic tarps and plastic tray liners. There was a full body suit inside along with a special pair of shoes to wear in her room.

When he completed the clean-room entrance, he knocked on the door and asked her if she needed anything other than liquids and food.

Eva responded, "No thanks. Just keep me hydrated and be careful, just in case."

"Okay. We are going to get you through this." He said before walking downstairs to start cooking her something to eat and getting her plenty of liquids. Randy was running low on bleach and needed to make a run to the market to buy some. Curfew only allowed people in his area to go out between five and eight in the morning, so he would have to wait for tomorrow.

When randy finished making her breakfast, he took the pancakes, scrambled eggs, and sausage up to her room and began his clean-room procedures. He set the tray of food and water down outside the entrance and began to remove his clothes. Once he was mostly stripped down he took the tray into the clean-room entrance. He set the tray down again and began to suit up with the gear he had brought up earlier.

He climbed into the pants, put on the long-sleeved shirt, put a mask over his mouth and nose, placed a pair of safety glasses over his eyes, pulled some shiny leather boots over his pants, and buttoned everything up before entering the room. He carried his bleach spray bottle with him and sprayed any surface he thought might contain remnants of bodily fluids or the virus.

The second he opened the door he asked, "How are you feeling, Eva?"

She was noticeably fatigued and replied, "I feel great, just a little tired. Nothing I won't get through in a day or two." Eva then forced a smile.

"You're going to be just fine." He guaranteed her as he took her the tray of food and water. "I've brought some extra snacks and water for you. I'll leave them on the end table for you."

Eva looked at him and said, "Don't get too close. I don't want you to catch the flu. I'll be fine. Just follow the plan." After she finished speaking, Eva put her head back down on the pillow and closed her eyes. "Thank you, Randy. I'll eat it in a little while."

He was hesitant to leave. "If you need anything at all, just call me. I'll be here for you."

As he made his way back out of the room, she said, "I will."

After closing the door to her room, he began to spray everything he was wearing with bleach-water. He paid particular attention to the soles of his shoes where a lot of things get stuck from walking around. After he sprayed bleach-water all over his clothes, and boots, he disrobed and sprayed his feet with the bleach solution before walking immediately to the bathroom for a shower with antibacterial soap.

Randy did the same thing several times over the course of the day. He spent a considerable amount of time thinking about what he could do to help her if she didn't get better. He decided he would make a call to her friend at the CDC if she wasn't better by tomorrow. Randy made his way to her room one more time to check on her before he went to sleep. She convinced him all was well and he went to bed.

January 26th, 2015

The first thing he thought of when he woke in the morning was Eva. He jumped up, ran to her wall, knocked, and said, "How you feeling this morning, Eva?"

She quietly responded, "Not very well. I've recently gotten diarrhea and started vomiting. I need you to bring me a thermometer and lots of fluids and soup."

He replied, "Hang in there, Eva. You're going to be just fine. I'm going to call your friend Larry at the CDC today and talk to him about what's happening."

"Okay." She muttered as she drifted back to sleep.

Randy went downstairs, made her breakfast, grabbed several bottles of water and a thermometer, and took it all to her. When he was done he went through the clean-room ordeal, showered, and went back downstairs to make the call to Larry at the CDC. He pulled the number from her phone.

Randy saved a copy of Larry's contact information in his phone for future reference. Eager and with nothing to lose, he dialed Larry on the phone.

It rang three times before he answered, "This is Dr. Larry Writer. Can I help you?"

Randy immediately seized the opportunity and said, "Larry, this is Randy, Eva's dear friend. She is showing symptoms and I'm very worried about her. You've been her friend for a little while now and I was hoping you could offer some of your expertise in her favor."

"I don't have any time to spare right now, so let's be quick about this." He said. "What symptoms is she showing?"

"She has fever, headache, chills, fatigue, diarrhea, abdominal pain, and she's vomiting." Randy told him.

There was a silence for several seconds before Larry began to speak again, "I'm sorry. Tell her I'm sorry. If those are her symptoms she could be gone before tomorrow morning. If her fever doesn't break I'm afraid she won't make it. I'm terribly sorry; I've got to get back to work." He said before hanging up the phone.

Randy fell back into the couch. This couldn't be. He looked to the heavens and angrily whispered under his breath, "Don't you even think about taking her. She is not finished with her work here, yet."

Then, he got up and walked back up to her room to tell her the news. "I've just gotten off the phone with Larry. He said you're going to be just fine." He fought back the tears as he said, "Yep, you're going to be just fine. I'm going to go do laundry. I'll check on you soon." Randy started at the door for a moment before walking down to the garage.

The second he had the garage door closed he sat down in the corner and cried. He begged and pleaded with god. "Whoever or whatever you are that has control over all that exists, please don't take her from me. She is all I have." He sat in silence for several minutes before standing up, wiping his eyes, and beginning to do some laundry.

When dinnertime came, he brought her food and a change of clothes. He went through the same cleaning and bleaching procedure every time he went into her room. Once he was finished for the evening, he retired to his and fell asleep.

January 27th, 2015

Randy woke to a fear he had not felt in his entire life. He rushed to her room and anxiously tapped on her wall, "Eva, how are you feeling?" He waited but got no answer. He hit the wall a little harder and said, "Eva, how are you feeling?" Again he waited in silence for a response. As he prepared to suit up and go in to check on her health, he heard her call from behind the wall. "Fever of 101.7, still vomiting, still have diarrhea, and still have all the other symptoms. I'm very weak. Bring me water and soup please."

He replied, "I was just going down to get us both something to eat and drink." Then he turned and walked down to the kitchen to make them both breakfast.

Randy returned about ten minutes later with a cold wet rag, some ibuprofen, soup, and ginger ale. Randy set them down outside of his little clean-room entrance, disrobed, and then stepped inside with the tray. He suited up like every other time and went inside.

"Hey Eva, how are you feeling?" He asked as soon as he was in the room.

"I think I've had better days." She said. "You should know how much I appreciate you taking care of me. A lot of people just cast people into the street when they show symptoms."

He cast a rapid rebuttal, "You are doing great and you'd take care of me too." Randy sat down next to her bed and gently rubbed her arm with his gloved hand. "I really do love you. I'd risk anything for you. You have to get better because I just realized how much you mean to me."

She tried to take it all in. Several moments passed before she responded, "I love you, too. However, I need more rest and less excitement. We will talk about it when I'm better."

He gently wiped her brow with the cold wet rag over and over so her fever would drop. To both of their surprise, her fever continued to climb. Hours went by and he became desperate when her fever hit 102.6 Fahrenheit. He tried more wet rags and ibuprofen, but nothing worked.

When her breath became shallow he knew they were near the end. He held her hand tight and ran his gloved fingers through her hair. Randy sat and told her of his love and the happy things they would someday do together.

It was completely unexpected when her fever suddenly broke and she began sweating. It dropped so rapidly that by the time he checked it again it had already lowered to 98.9 Fahrenheit. This meant she would likely live. Randy was left alone to experience the thrill of knowing she would live as Eva had finally fallen asleep for the night.

Randy made his way out of the room and cleaned his clothes and himself like always. When he finally finished for the day, he made himself a small dinner and ate it in his room before he went to sleep.

That night Randy dreamed of a new beginning with happiness and joy throughout the entire world. Sadly, his dream had a lot of pain and horror in store for the world before it could turn into bliss. Luckily, he didn't believe in the power of dreams.

February 18th, 2015

Eva may have survived, but that was not the case for the 90% of people who died from being infected during the hibernation period. Even the national and international headlines were bleak. 'Three Million Dead' covered the front of every paper.

This outbreak turned into a plague that took hold of everyone who fell within its' grasp. The experts who are still alive have said the outbreak could reach critical mass sometime in the next three months. If we fail to contain the spread like we have to this point, not many people will survive. They also believe at the current rate we will have lost nearly 20% of the global population to Ebola before November 15th, 2015.

Randy and Eva tightened up their overall security, but everything else remained about the same. They both acted like the incident where they 'confessed their love' didn't even happen. Things went on relatively normal for life during the epidemic that was wiping out the globe.

After waking up and checking his email, the news, and social media, Randy told Eva the virus had spread to another quarter of a million people.

She replied, "I spoke to Larry yesterday. He said they are on the verge of another possible cure. If everything goes well, we could have one ready for everyone that is infected before June of this year."

"That's great news!" He exclaimed. "Maybe humanity can survive this after-all."

"I sure hope so." Eva said. "You know we need to go out there and get groceries today, right?"

Randy quietly said, "I've seen the pantry. We need a lot of things. I'll suit up and head to the store after we have lunch."

"I don't mean to force you to go out there. If something happened to you it would devastate me." She told him.

"There isn't much contact out there between people anymore." He replied. "If someone is walking around without protective gear it is safe to assume they are a contagious carrier."

She fired back, "I don't want you becoming one of them. We need to both live through this thing. That is final."

Randy smiled, "You got it boss. Just write me a list of things we need." Then he flipped through the television channels while she wrote him a list of things they needed.

She finished the list and gave it to him before he had a chance to settle on any one television show. "Here is the list." She said. "Stay cautious. I got sick while being careful.

Things are more dangerous now and more deadly. Don't go getting yourself sick like I did. I can't do this alone."

"You won't have to. I'll be fine." He replied. "I'll suit up and head out to the market before curfew kicks in." He headed into the garage and went through the process of covering his body with protective materials to help him keep infected fluids off of his body and out of his system. On his way out the garage door he grabbed his bleach spray bottle and his hand sanitizer.

When he got to the store everyone was wearing what appeared to be hazmat suits. The employees were all in their own sealed boxes wearing protective equipment. Apparently, this was the only way to keep the supply chain open for everyone.

Randy walked through the store and picked up the things they had in stock, tried to substitute the ones they didn't, and added a few other things in for good measure. After paying for his groceries, he headed home. The street was extremely empty. All the lights were green. Most businesses were closed, some temporary, some permanent. It was very humbling.

When he got home, Randy entered the garage and went through the cleaning stages for the food, his clothes, and himself. Then he put the groceries away and sat down to watch a movie with Eva. She was so bored she fell asleep in the middle of the show. No more than two minutes later Randy followed her into a deep slumber.

Waking up in each others arms had become somewhat commonplace. Still, nothing had happened between the two of them. At least, nothing had happened, yet. There was certainly an air of tension forming between them.

June 8th, 2015

The sun was shining in his window, but Randy had lost his drive to jump right out of bed. Instead, he stayed still as the sunlight shone into his eyes. It seemed to take hours to build up the energy, but the clock only turned the hands of time by seven minutes. When he opened his door the smell of food cooking in the kitchen hit him like a Christmas morning breakfast at Grandma's house. He was drawn down to the table.

Eva was waiting for him in the kitchen. She had gotten up early to make them breakfast. "I checked the news this morning." She said as she turned the eggs in the pan.

He paused for a moment, wondering if he should ask what she read. "You might as well come out with it. Is it good or bad?"

Eva brought two plates of food to the table and sat down. "Well, there is good and bad. The good news is that the trials for the new cure have shown positive results. All patients that have received the new drug have survived. They are going to quarantine them for three weeks now and ensure no side effects like the last big inoculation."

Randy took a bite of his food and nodded in agreement at the good news.

She continued, "The bad news is the infection is spreading faster than before. There are now over 600,000,000 people thought to be infected. The latest numbers show over 200,000,000 people have already died. We are not out of the woods yet."

He responded, "If we can just stay here and make sure we don't bring the virus home, we should be able to survive."

"That's not all" She told him. "The utilities and supply chain have been failing in Western nations around the world. It could happen here, too."

"I guess it's a good thing I upgraded to solar power a few years ago and had a deepwater well dug out back." He said. "We just need to make sure we have enough food to last us through this."

"Speaking of which…" She said. "I'm going to go to town for more bleach and supplies. We are running low on canned foods."

Randy said, "You know, the only grocer left open is Randal's on sixth and main. It's going to be very busy. Do you want me to go with you?"

"No." Eva responded. "There is no reason to risk you becoming infected. I didn't think I was going to live through my ordeal. Besides, I have less risk because I survived once already."

"The virus could have mutated by now." He argued. "That was months ago. You still need to take every precaution."

She replied, "I will. Write me a list of things to get. I'll pick up what I can. Now, finish your breakfast."

When they were done, he wrote a list and she began getting suited up in the garage. She covered her body from head to toe and made sure she had a small spray bottle of bleach-water and a bottle of hand sanitizer.

He watched out the window as she drove off, turned to his computer, and started working on the next chapter of his latest book. After-all, the income from his books is what allowed them to stay at home the majority of the time. Without it, they would be forced to have a regular job and risk likely infection.

Randy began to get worried after Eva had been gone for over an hour. They always kept the trips to the grocer under an hour to minimize risk of contamination. She had been gone now for over an hour and a half.

When she finally arrived he was so happy that he didn't even question how long she was gone. He couldn't have even if he had wanted to. She immediately started telling him what happened while she was out. "It's getting really bad out there, Randy. There were sick people walking, laying, and dying in the streets. I ran into a government truck picking them up for quarantine in some camp they have setup outside of town. The grocer was having trouble getting most of their stock through the supply chain, so all I could get was rice, beans, potatoes, and a few cans of spam. Let me get clean and I'll tell you the rest inside."

"I'll meet you in the living room." He told her as he walked inside the house. Once she had finished and come inside she met him on the couch. He could tell she was distraught.

"It was the most horrible thing I've ever seen." Eva told him as tears began to roll down her face. "They were forcing everyone that had a fever into the back of these military trucks." She paused and put her hands on her face to cry, "I watched them shoot a man who refused to get in the truck. It was so scary."

Randy put his arm around her and said, "Don't worry. Everything is going to be okay. You're home now. We'll find out what's going on and figure it out."

She replied, "I don't think it's going to be that easy. We must keep a low profile from now on. I am not going to wind up in some camp and neither are you."

"Okay, I promise we won't wind up in some camp." He reassured her.

They spent the rest of the night lying on the couch watching old shows. Nothing eventful happened the rest of the evening and they once again passed out in each others arms.

September 12th, 2015

When Eva hung up the phone she looked at Randy with a blank stare. She didn't know how to tell him.

He eagerly asked, "What happened? What's wrong? Did the cure fail?"

"No." She replied. "Larry died last week. They think he did it, but not in time to save himself. I think there's a cure!"

"Let's not jump to conclusions." He quickly chimed in. "We should wait to hear about it on the news."

She replied, "Yes, certainly. We will wait to hear about it on the news. The man I spoke with said they would be doing an emergency broadcast tonight at 8:37PM."

He was confused, "8:37PM? Not 8:30PM?"

"Something about not looking planned." Eva told him.

They ate lunch and waited for the broadcast at 8:37PM. When it came on they were glued to the TV.

The Broadcast said, "This is a broadcast to the people of the United States of America. While we have lost many wonderful people including Dr Larry Writer, the scientist behind the cure, we are now ready to fight back. We have a tested cure for this strain of Ebola. We are ready to begin inoculations immediately. The direst of cases within government quarantine centers will be the first to be administered the cure. From there we will go down the list to those in most need until we have inoculated the entire population. The CDC is working with governments around the world to ensure global inoculation. We urge people to remain calm during this time and stay indoors. If you would like to report a severe case of Ebola, please call 1-800-INFO-NOW."

When the message began to repeat itself they both stood up and started dancing. It looked sort of like a rain dance, but without a fire, and they didn't have drums.

He repeated, "We're going to live. We're going to live. We are going to live!"

She interjected, "Wait. We can't get our hopes up that high just yet. This could still fail. Remember last time."

"You're right." He replied. "But at least we can start planning for it to be over. This nightmare we've faced for almost a year now. It could have become a lot worse."

"Worse?" She asked. "Did you forget the death toll is over eight hundred million people? There's more than a billion people currently infected. People with Ebola have been treating people with Ebola. That's how bad it is, Randy."

"You're right." He said. "I'm sorry. I didn't mean to make light of what has already happened. This virus is the most devastating thing we've experienced in all of recorded history."

Eva dropped back on to the couch and said, "Either way, it doesn't matter. Things might get better and might not."

He replied, "I sure hope things get better." Then he headed off into his room to work on his book.

October 23rd, 2015

Eva called out, "Randy, the President's on the TV. Come quick, he's talking about the inoculation."

As he was getting up he said, "Be right there."

When he reached the living room he sat down on the couch next to Eva. They stared at the TV and waited for him to begin. It was a trancelike moment.

While they waited it became apparent his beard had grown out since he stopped shaving and she had forgone shaving and wearing nice clothes. They looked like a young homely couple.

Suddenly, the President walked out onto the screen and started speaking, "My fellow Americans and citizens of the world. Today is a day that will forever go down in history as the day we extinguished the epidemic that stole from us nearly 18% of the people on earth." He paused for a moment. "There is not a human being alive today who has not lost a brother, a sister, a mother, a father, a lover, a friend, or a child. We have suffered so much, but the worst is now behind us. We have inoculated all those who showed symptoms or had been exposed. It is time for humanity to rebuild. We will come together to create a more powerful society that is engineered around the true threats to a modern world. We will spread out and work toward carbon neutrality. Humanity will work together for the betterment of all life on earth, for as the earth thrives, humanity thrives. Together, we will seize the opportunity - in this tragedy - to form a tighter bond with our neighbors, our friends, our allies, and especially our enemies. Humanity will get through this.

Power and all other necessary utilities have been being restored all over the world. Within weeks we will be functioning at nearly 60% what we were at our peak. This is your time now." The President again pauses for a moment. "Tomorrow, at 5:00AM the curfew will be lifted. I encourage you and all people around the globe to go back to work. United we stand as one people of earth. Good night and God Bless."

When the President finished speaking the screen went blank. Randy and Eva turned to each other and at the same time said, "Did you hear that?" Then they both said, "You go."

Randy paused long enough for Eva to say, "That means I can go back to work! I've been cooped up here for a little too long." She stopped, looked at Randy, and said, "I don't want to move out. This means we can be together." When she finished talking she watched him and waited for a reaction.

He didn't hesitate, "I love you, Eva. I've always loved you. It's been killing me to be so close, but so far away. I don't want to let you out of my sight."

"Then don't." She said. "Let me move in here. We can take things slow at first. It won't be much different than it's been for nearly the last year. I'll just stay instead of move back to my place."

"Okay." He said. "I'm game. Why wouldn't I be? I just told you, I love you."

"I think I love you, too." She confessed as she leaned in for a kiss. Magic shot through their bodies when their lips met.

They didn't know if it was the adrenaline from the news, the lips of one another, or something else, but it didn't matter in the end, the only thing that mattered was how they both felt when they were together. They spent the next few days in each others arms. For a little while they were able to become so lost in each others arms that they completely forgot about the virus and the suffering outside their walls.

October 26th, 2015

Randy opened his eyes to see Eva lying next to him. Everything felt so right. It was almost too good to be true, but here it was, happening. The alarm buzzer started going off and he hit the snooze and nudged Eva lightly, "Eva, sweetheart, it's time to get up for work."

She rolled over and said, "I'm getting up." Then she fell back asleep.

Again he gently shook her and said, "Baby, you need to wake up for work."

This time she sat up and opened one eye. When she saw him she immediately smiled and gave him a kiss. Eva climbed out of bed and got ready to go out for her day meeting new clients. They have been lining up for months. Some of them she was able to handle from home, but most need a personal meeting with her.

Randy went downstairs and made her a full breakfast complete with pancakes, eggs, hash browns, sausage, bacon, and toast. Right as the toast popped up she sat down at the table. He dropped a plate full of food in front of her and one in front of himself. They both flirted rather quietly while they ate their breakfast.

She said, "Wish me luck with these new clients today, honey."

"Good luck, Eva." He said as she was walking out the front door. No protective suit. No garage routine with bleach and washing machines. He realized at that moment they were getting back to normalcy like the President said.

They waved at each other as she started backing out the driveway. He stepped back inside and closed the door before heading to the computer to continue working on his book. He thought to himself, "What an incredibly exhausting and horrifying journey we just ended."

He picked up a soda and took a sip before placing his hands on the keyboard and writing his next book like it was all just a bad dream.

Tips to stay Safe

#1

Ebola is a virus spread through bodily fluids like blood, vomit, feces, urine, sweat, semen, and saliva. Stay clean and don't get any of these fluids into an open wound, your eyes, your mouth, or any other orifice.

#2

Humans are contagious when they are showing symptoms. They can be contagious after death, so be weary of any bodily fluids or corpses. Keep your body clean of fluids and keep your body covered.

#3

Bleach is your best friend. Bleach kills Ebola on contact and is used extensively in West African nations to combat the spread of Ebola. Using a spray bottle or some other method, mist or saturate surfaces in bleach to ensure they are completely sanitized.

#4

Ebola is not airborne as of this writing and therefore is only a threat if you touch the physical bodily fluids of someone who is infected. You will not catch Ebola from breathing the same air as someone with the virus.

#5

To lower the risk of possible infection, clean your hands regularly with antibacterial soaps and hand sanitizer. This can help eliminate Ebola from the surface of your hand before it is accidentally spread to your body.

#6

Ebola rarely lives longer than 24 hours on a dry surface outside of a host. Though, the virus can live several days at room temperature *inside of liquid or bodily fluids. Most low traffic areas will be of lower risk for infection contamination because of this.*

#7

The World Health Organization says Ebola can spread through the semen of a survivor for as long as seven weeks after being declared cured.

#8

Burying or incinerating the bodies of the deceased is the quickest way to ensure they can't spread the virus further. Many aid workers in hot-zones also choose to bury or burn their protective equipment with the body.

#9

The easiest way to survive Ebola is to stay out of the outbreak zones and have quality cleaning procedures for anyone who enters the living residence. In the story, we spoke about the garage with the washing machine, large sink, and shower for cleaning off before entering the house.

#10

Stocking up on supplies while they are available is a good way to survive any disaster. In the event of an epidemic, you will probably want to have anywhere from six months to two years worth of food. You will also need a long term sustainable food plan.

#11

Be prepared to shelter in place for the long term. You need to have enough supplies to be able to survive alone for months at a time. Some people prepare for years off the grid.

#12

A chlorine solution of 0.5% available chlorine is best for sanitizing surfaces and other things from Ebola. If properly used, chlorine bleach is extremely effective at combating Ebola. There are many other sanitizers available that can kill Ebola.

Thanks for reading

If you enjoyed the book or thought you learned from it at all, please go online and let everyone know how much you enjoyed it with a review.

It isn't easy to let people know what to expect from a book you wrote, but with reviews they get a good idea.

Thanks for reading. I hope you enjoyed the story and learned something.